The Complete
BODY MOISTURIZER
GUIDE FOR
BEGINNERS

Natural Body Butter Recipes for Rejuvenating and Hydrating your Skin

EVA HUNTER

Table of Contents

Introduction

I want to thank you and congratulate you for purchasing the book, *"BODY MOISTURIZER GUIDE FOR BEGINNERS: Natural Body Butter Recipes for Rejuvenating and Hydrating your Skin"*.

This book contains proven steps and strategies on how to keep your skin healthy and radiant with all natural body butter recipes that you can make right at home.

You've seen those brands before, luxury skin care brands that sell overpriced body butters that are supposed to give your skin the nourishment it needs. While the latter is true, the price certainly isn't reasonable for the Average Jane. But don't fret! In this eBook, we'll provide you with what you need to know about body butters as well as different easy to follow recipes that are sure to get you started on the right foot when it comes to making some of your own.

Thanks again for purchasing this book, I hope you enjoy it! Please take some time to stop by and LIKE our Facebook page:

https://www.facebook.com/joypublishing

With gratitude,

EVA HUNTER

Chapter 1: The Benefits of Natural Body Butters

What exactly are body butters? Aren't they just "glorified" lotions and basically do the same things as your basic one? To help you better understand, here's a quick rundown of everything you need to know about body butter along with the different benefits that you could derive from it.

Body butters are basically nutrient dense creams that are meant to hydrate the skin to the fullest; much more than your average lotion. Typically, body butters also make use of all natural ingredients such as cocoa butter, coconut oil, mango butter as well as Shea butter. By themselves, these ingredients can bring a number of great benefits for your skin. Below, you'll find a quick list.

Cocoa Butter

Lightens Stretch Marks - It has been widely noted that this can help in reducing stretch marks; many pregnant women all over the world would rub this on their bellies to help lessen the appearance of stretch marks as well as to keep their skin healthy throughout the pregnancy itself. Besides stretch marks, it can also trigger faster skin healing for certain scars that may have darkened over time.

Antioxidants - It also contains a high amount of antioxidants that help in fighting off free radicals. These free radicals are the most common causes of skin aging as well as different skin issues such as acne.

Deep Hydration - This is especially important when it comes to the colder seasons wherein our skin tends to get flaky due to the lack of moisture. Because cocoa butter contains a high amount of fatty acids, it is able to hydrate our skin thoroughly and deeply.

Shea Butter

Skin Super Food - Shea butter is known to be moisturizing as well as skin regenerating. It can help protect your skin from UV sunlight and at the same time, provide ample hydration when the climates get harsh. Aside from these, it can also help strengthen your skin by stimulating your skin's ability to produce collagen-- which makes it great for anti-aging as well. It would make your skin more supple and give it that healthy, radiant glow.

Healing - Because Shea butter also has anti-inflammatory and healing attributes, it can also contribute to treating certain skin problems and disorders such as: psoriasis, eczema, rashes (especially diaper ones), insect bites, hives, skin cracks, minor burns and cuts, dermatitis caused by contact with poisonous plants and even sunburn when you have spent too much time out in the heat. It is very calming and soothing on the skin which helps in easing any of the discomfort caused by any of the above.

Besides this, its benefits can go beyond skin deep. In fact, men and women who do a lot of sports could benefit a lot from getting regular massages using Shea butter. It helps the muscles recover faster and better. At the same time, it also helps reduce muscle aches and eliminates toxins from their overworked muscles.

Coconut Oil

Moisturizing - Often, people would use a couple of skin moisturizers when it comes to their skin. One for hydration and the other to help fight against skin-aging. With coconut oil, you won't need anything else for it has components that would tackle both of those. The best bit? It also contains anti-bacterial properties that means that it could help you with acne problems as well; something that you would not typically expect from an oil.

It is known to be deeply moisturizing, providing your skin with all the nutrients that it needs to stay healthy as well as strengthen collagen production thus helping you keep that youthful glow. For people who enjoy going to the beach but want something that would protect their skin from the UV rays, this is also great for that purpose and used in conjunction with other ingredients such as Shea butter. It only gets better.

Treating Skin Disorders - Much like Shea butter, it also known to be very helpful when it comes to the treatment of eczema and psoriasis. It does this by killing of the microbial bodies that are often the cause of these issues-- at the same time, it heals the broken skin by stimulating the growth of healthy skin cells. So if these skin disorders have left visible marks on your skin, such as acne scars, using coconut oil regularly would help fade those away.

Mango Butter

Anti-Aging - When it comes to anti-aging, mango butter is one of the most potent ingredients that you can add to body butters. It is highly effective when it comes to rejuvenating the skin simply because it contains a generous amount of antioxidants. These antioxidants help in neutralizing the toxins in our skin and at the same time, promote cell renewal which also prevents the formation of wrinkles, fine lines and other skin issues that are brought on by aging.

Mango butter contains a lot of valuable skin acids as well; among which are, stearic acid, oleic acid and linoleic acid. Aside from these, it also contains vitamin A as well as a high amount of vitamin E, D and C along with calcium, folic acid, magnesium and iron. All of which are great for the skin's overall appearance and health. Lastly, it is also capable of protecting your skin from sun damage.

Chapter 2: The Benefits of Different Essential Oils

In the recipes that you will be provided with, you might notice the frequent use of different essential oils. In this chapter, we will look more into their uses and the benefits that they add to our body butters.

Cinnamon - It contains anti-fungal, antibacterial, astringent, antimicrobial, anti-clotting, cooling and carminative properties. As for the benefits, it is frequently used as a brain tonic-- but is more known for being able to treat certain respiratory problems, different skin infections along with healing wounds. Cinnamon can also be used to improve any blood impurity and circulation issues, as well as provide relief for pain including menstrual problems.

Grapefruit - This is a known disinfectant, antiseptic, tonic, diuretic and stimulant. For the skin, it provides a layer of protection from different infections. If you have acne scars or just light scars in general, it can help lighten it by eliminating any of the toxin built up on your skin. It is also often used as an aromatherapy oil so if you use it before bed, you will certainly benefit from its ability to bring you better and easier sleep.

Jasmine - This is a known antiseptic and aphrodisiac. For the skin, it can help protect wounds as well as heal scars along with different after marks. So if you have certain spots on your skin or unevenness, regularly using body butter that's been infused with jasmine would certainly help. It is also capable of uplifting your mood and works as an effective aromatherapy product.

Lavender - This is among the most commonly used essential oil mostly because of its aromatherapy benefits which can easily calm you down and help in removing the stress from your muscles.

Other than that, lavender is also very soothing and relaxing--especially if you are using it for skin issues such as sunburn or even minor burns. It hastens the skin's ability to heal and relieves any discomfort associated with different skin problems.

Lemon - Another commonly used essential oil when it comes to body butter's thanks to its refreshing scent as well as astringent and antiviral properties. It helps in protecting your skin from bacteria along with helping in lightening any scars that you have. It is especially effective when it comes to dealing with acne scars as well as minor wounds that might have left marks on your skin. As for skin health, it promotes firmness and slows aging down.

Peppermint - Typically used as a decongestant or even as an expectorant, peppermint has quite a lot of surprising skin health benefits that you should take advantage of. To begin with, it helps in relaxing your muscles and promoting skin as well as muscle repair. So if you are on the sporty side and working out is a regular part of your day, going home and massaging yourself with body butter infused with peppermint would help detoxify your skin as well as promote healing. It also firms the skin up, making it look more youthful and rejuvenated.

Rose - Roses are quite high in vitamin C and are very potent antioxidants. It is capable of protecting your skin from sun damage as well as provide relief should you experience sunburn. It is also one of the more moisturizing essential oils, able to go deep into your skin and effectively rehydrate it. This is something that would certainly come in handy during the colder months or even on a daily basis, if you spent a lot of your time outdoors.

Tea Tree - If you have skin issues such as acne or pigmentation, tea tree oil would be the best remedy for those. It is a known antimicrobial, antiseptic, antimicrobial and antiviral. It can help protect wounds as well as speed up the healing period for different scars as well as after marks. It is also capable of clearing acne.

Rosemary - This helps in rejuvenating our skin as well as hydrating it properly. If you have been experiencing unevenness in your skin tone, this also works with that. Rosemary essential oil also contains anti-aging properties that can help bring back the firmness of your skin, making it appear younger and lessen the appearance of fine lines. Its regenerative properties promote healing and replacement of any damaged tissue. Lastly, it is also another effective acne treatment-- able to remove the acne itself and fade out any leftover scars after.

Chapter 3: Skin Moisturizing Body Butters

Magnesium Body Butter

Ingredients:

- 3 tablespoons of Shea Butter
- 2 tablespoons of beeswax (in pastille form)
- ½ cup of magnesium flakes along with 3 tablespoons of boiling water (You can also make use of pre-made magnesium oil, however, this won't yield the same amount of magnesium when it comes to the final product)
- ¼ cup of unrefined coconut oil

Procedure:

1. Add your boiling water to the magnesium flakes, stirring until it dissolves completely. This should create a thick liquid. Set this aside to cool while you work on the other ingredients.

2. In a mason jar or heat safe bowl, melt your beeswax, coconut oil and Shea butter together using a double boiler. Keep the heat on medium or low.

3. Once melted, remove the jar from the heat and allow it to cool. This should firm up within half an hour and the color should change to something opaque.

4. Once cool enough to touch, blend it using an immersion or hand blender using medium speed. Slowly, add your

melted magnesium into mix. Once done, put this in the fridge for 15 minutes before blending again.

5. You should get a nice body butter consistency after-- but you can make it as thick or thin as you wish by adding more   coconut   oil.   Store   it   in   the   fridge.

Lavender Infused Body Butter

Ingredients:

- 10 drops of lavender essential oil
- 4 tablespoons of coconut oil
- 2 tablespoons of beeswax
- 15 tablespoons of olive oil
- 1 teaspoon of honey
- 2 teaspoons of lanolin
- 3 tablespoons of aloe vera gel
- 1 vitamin e capsule

Procedure:

1. Following the steps from the previous recipe, melt your beeswax together with your oils in a double boiler. Once melted, add your honey into the mix and stir slowly until it gets incorporated well.

2. In a separate double boiler, heat your aloe before adding it into your beeswax mixture. Stir slowly then add your lanolin as well.

3. Once everything has combined, lower your heat and add your Vitamin E as well as lavender essential oil. Take this off of the heat and allow it to cool.

4. Once firmer, whip until it becomes smooth. Store it in a cool place.

Rosemary Infused Body Butter

Ingredients:

- 10 drops of rosemary essential oil
- 90 grams of Shea butter
- 45 grams of cocoa butter
- 20 drops of spearmint essential oil
- 45 grams of kukui nut oil

Procedure:

1. Using the double boiler method, melt your Shea and cocoa butter together. Stir slowly while you add the rest of your oils.

2. Once incorporated properly, remove this from the heat and refrigerate for a few minutes or until it turns opaque and slightly solid-- but not too much. Make sure that it does not completely solidify or you will have to melt it again.

3. Get your hand mixer or an immersion blender and whip this mixture up to your desired consistency. You can add more kukui nut oil as needed but remember that this will make your body butter a bit thinner than most.

4. Store in a cool place.

Vanilla and Coconut Oil Body Butter

Ingredients:

- 1 cup of coconut oil
- 1 teaspoon of vitamin oil
- a few drops of vanilla infused oil
- A teaspoon of honey

Procedure:

1. Put all of your ingredients in a mixing bowl. You do not have to melt your coconut oil for this one and if you are working with one that is liquid, keep it in the fridge for a few minutes to make it solidify a bit.

2. Mix your ingredients thoroughly before you take out the mixer.

3. Whip your mixture for at least 5 minutes or up until it begins to peak, resembling whip cream only firmer and a lot more delicious smelling.

4. Transfer this to your container and store in a cool place.

Mango and Citrus Body Butter

Ingredients:

- 10 grams of jojoba wax or beeswax
- 25 grams of cocoa butter
- 25 grams of mango butter
- 30 grams of Shea butter
- 1 teaspoon of almond oil
- 1 teaspoon of vitamin e
- 15 drops of citrus essential oil (you can add more or reduce the amount depending on your own preferences)

Procedure:

1. Begin by melting your mango butter, beeswax and cocoa butter using a double boiler. Keep your heat low and let it sit on that for about 15 to 20 minutes. This would help prevent your butter from becoming grainy once it cools.

2. Once completely melted, add in your vitamin E and almond oil. Stir these in gently.

3. Remove it from the heat and while still hot, add your essential oils. Stir it thoroughly.

4. Allow this to cool down for a few minutes before transferring it to your container where it would completely set.

Coconut Rose Body Butter

Ingredients:

- 60 grams of refined coconut oil
- 10 drops of rose essential oil
- 10 grams of jojoba oil
- 3 grams cornstarch
- 1 ml alkanet infused oil

Procedure:

1. Mix your alkanet infused oil, jojoba oil, coconut oil and cornstarch in a heat safe bowl then place it in your double boiler.

2. Mix everything well until the coconut oil melts completely.

3. Take it off of the heat and allow it to cool at room temp.

4. Add in your essential oils and whisk until it becomes fluffy or gets to the consistency of frosting.

5. Transfer it to your sanitized container and store in a cool place.

Shea Butter and Honey Body Butter

Ingredients:

- 1 cup of organic raw Shea butter
- 1 tablespoon of organic honey
- ½ cup of almond oil
- ½ cup of coconut oil
- Your favorite essential oil

Procedure:

1. Using a double boiler, melt your Shea butter thoroughly. Once done, take it off of the heat and stir in your honey. Let this sit for about half an hour.

2. Stir in your almond oil and your chosen essential oil.

3. Put it in the freezer until your oils starts to firm up again or gets opaque. This should allow you to whip it better.

4. Using a hand mixer or even an immersion blender, whip it for a few minutes until it begins to peak or forms a frosting like consistency.

5. Keep in a clean jar and store in a cool place.

Chapter 4: Healing and Skin Protection Body Butters

Anti-winter Dryness Body Butter

Ingredients:

- 2 cups of organic coconut oil
- 7 ounces of Shea butter
- 1 drop of tea tree oil
- And your choice of essential oil (recommended: lavender and peppermint)

Procedure:

1. Using a double boiler, melt your coconut oil and Shea butter until it liquefies. Remove this from your heat and add the essential oils along with your tea tree oil. Stir well.

2. Allow this to cool. You can also pop it into the fridge for 10 to 15 minutes. Once it turns opaque and slightly firm, you can take it out.

3. Get your mixer and start whipping up the mixture until it peaks or reaches the consistency of frosting or butter.

4. Store in a cool place to extend shelf life.

Cinnamon Body Butter to Prevent Cellulite

Ingredients:

- 50 grams of cocoa butter
- 100 grams of coconut oil
- 50 grams of Shea butter
- A cinnamon stick
- 30 drops of cinnamon oil

Procedure:

1. Bring out the double boiler and over low heat, slowly melt your Shea butter as well as your coconut oil if yours has solidified. Keep it on the heat until both become liquid.

2. Remove it from the heat after and allow it to cool for at least 10 to 20 minutes. Don't put it in the fridge, let it set slowly.

3. Add your cinnamon oil after it cools down a bit.

4. Whip it until the texture becomes fluffy and light. At this point break off pieces of your cinnamon stick and add it to your mixture. Mix well.

5. Store in an air tight container and keep somewhere cool.

Vitamin E Oil Body Butter

Ingredients:

- ¼ Coconut Oil
- ½ cup of Shea Butter
- ½ teaspoon Vanilla Oil
- 1 tablespoon of Vitamin E Oil

Procedure:

Melt your coconut oil and Shea butter over low heat using your double boiler. Make sure to stir it gently so everything gets mixed together well.

1. Once melted, remove it from the heat and let it sit for at least 20 minutes before adding your vanilla oil. Stir again and then add your vitamin E oil. Mix well.

2. Place this mixture in the fridge for half an hour or until it turns opaque and becomes slightly firm.

3. Take it out of your fridge and using a hand mixer, whip it up until it peaks and reaches the consistency of frosting. Remember that the more you whip, the fluffier it gets.

4. Store in a clean container and keep in a cool place.

Refreshing Peppermint Body Butter

Ingredients:

- 2 oz. of cocoa butter
- 6 oz. of coconut oil
- Peppermint essential oil

Procedure:

1. Melt your cocoa butter and coconut oil over low heat using your double boiler. Make sure it is melted well. Don't forget to stir slowly.

2. Take it off of the heat and let it sit for a few minutes before adding your essential oil. Stir some more.

3. Bring out your whisk or hand mixer and start whipping. Do this for 5 to 10 minutes or until you get the consistency that you prefer.

4. Store in a sanitized jar and keep somewhere cool for a longer shelf life.

Black Raspberry and Vanilla Body Butter

Ingredients:

- 156 grams of cocoa butter
- 24 grams of grape seed oil
- 155 grams of Shea butter
- 65 grams of apricot kernel oil
- 4 grams vitamin e oil
- 10 grams raspberry vanilla fragrance oil

Procedure:

1. Begin with melting all of your butters properly by using a double boiler. Stir gently until everything gets mixed.

2. Once melted, remove it from the heat and let it sit for a few minutes before adding your essential oil and your vitamin E oil. Stir gently again.

3. Allow this to cool for a few minutes. You can also place it in the fridge to hasten the process.

4. Once it becomes opaque and is slightly firm to the touch, you can start whipping. Using your hand mixer or a whisk, whip the mixture for 10 to 15 minutes. It should become the consistency of frosting but if it doesn't, place it back in the fridge for a few more minutes before trying again.

5. Once done, transfer to a clean container and store in some place cool.

Anti-Bacterial Body Butter

Ingredients:

- ½ cup of coconut oil
- 2 tablespoons of jojoba oil
- 6 tablespoons of cocoa butter
- A couple drops of progest E (you can add more if desired)
- 15 drops of tea tree oil (you can increase the amount but be sure to do a spot test first to make sure you are not too sensitive to it)
- Your favorite essential oil

Procedure:

1. Using your double boiler, melt your cocoa butter slowly over low heat. Make sure it does not get too hot. Once melted, remove it from the heat.

2. At this point, slowly stir in your coconut oil, essential oil and jojoba oil. Mix all three well and let it sit, allowing it to solidify. You can also place it in the fridge the speed up the process.

3. Once somewhat solid, take out your mixer and whip it for a good 10 or so minutes. Add your tea tree oil and stir it into the mix before whipping it once more.

4. Store in a clean container and keep some place cool.

Vanilla Bean Body Butter

Ingredients:

- 1 vanilla bean
- 1 cup of raw cocoa butter
- ½ cup of coconut oil
- ½ cup of sweet almond oil

Procedure:

1. Melt your cocoa butter and coconut together using a double boiler over low heat. Give this about 30 minutes and gently stir it ever so often.

2. Once melted, take it off of the heat and stir in your sweet almond oil into the mixture.

3. Grind your vanilla bean and add this to the mix.

4. Place the mixture in your freezer for about 20 minutes, allowing the oils to slightly solidify.

5. Once ready, take it out of the fridge and whip it until the texture reaches a thick frosting like consistency.

6. Transfer to a clean container and store it some place cold.

Chapter 5: Refreshing and Skin Nourishing Body Butters

Coconut Oil Cooling Body Butter

Ingredients:

- 1 cup of coconut oil
- ½ cup of aloe gel
- 18 drops of essential oils (lavender or peppermint would work best)

Procedure:

1. Put all of your ingredients in a mixing bowl. Mix them first with a spoon.

2. After, take out your mixer or a whisk and start whipping the mixture. Do this for about 5 to 10 minutes depending on how long it takes for it to peak.

3. Once done, scoop it all into a clean container and keep some place cool to prolong its shelf life.

Bronzing Body Butter (Extra Nourishing)

Ingredients:

- 1 cup of Shea butter
- ½ cup of olive oil
- ½ cup of coconut oil
- 1-2 tablespoons of cacao powder
- 1 tablespoon ground nutmeg
- 2 tablespoons of vitamin E oil
- 2 tablespoons ground cinnamon
- 8 drops of your preferred essential oil

Procedure:

1. Using your double boiler, melt your Shea butter together with your coconut oil. Once completely liquefied, remove it from the heat and let it cool for about half an hour.

2. Add your cacao powder, olive oil, nutmeg, cinnamon, Vitamin E and your chosen essential oil. Stir well and make sure everything gets mixed properly.

3. Place in the fridge until it firms up slightly.

4. Take it out of the fridge and using your mixer, whip the mixture until it peaks. It should be the consistency of frosting or whipped butter.

5. Transfer this into a clean container and store somewhere cool.

Mint Chocolate Whipped Butter

Ingredients:

- ½ cup of organic cocoa butter
- ½ cup of organic mango butter
- ½ cup of jojoba oil
- ½ cup of coconut oil
- 1 to 2 teaspoons of peppermint essential oil
- 2 tablespoons of cacao powder
- 2 teaspoons of vitamin E

Procedure:

1. Begin with the usual, melting your butters and oils using a double boiler until it becomes completely liquid. Once done, remove it from the heat.

2. Let this sit for 10 to 15 minutes before adding the rest of your ingredients to the mix, making sure that you stir everything well so that it gets incorporated properly.

3. Keep this in your fridge for half an hour or up until it starts to slightly solidify. That should make whipping much easier.

4. Once firm, whip it for around 10 minutes or up until the mixture begins to peak. Depending on the consistency you want, you can continue whipping the mix.

5. Store in an airtight jar and keep somewhere cool.

Creamy Mango Body Butter

Ingredients:

- 2/3 cup of Shea butter
- 1 teaspoon of jojoba oil
- 1/3 cup of mango butter
- 2 teaspoons of grapeseed oil
- ¼ teaspoon of vitamin e oil
- 8 drops of lemongrass essential oil
- 1 teaspoon of cornstarch (to lessen the oily feel)

Procedure:

1. To get started, melt both your butters using a double boiler while keeping the heat low. Stir this gently to mix them and once melted thoroughly, remove it from the heat.

2. Let this sit for at least 15 minutes until it cools down a bit before you add the rest of your ingredients. Mix properly and make sure that the cornstarch gets dissolved completely.

3. Keep this in the fridge for at least 20 minutes or until it becomes somewhat firmer and ready for mixing.

4. Once it gets to that stage, take it out and start whipping. Remember that the more you whip, the fluffier and lighter it will get. So it all depends on your preferences and what you're looking for.

5. Store in a sanitized container and keep somewhere cool to lengthen shelf life.

Conclusion

Thank you again for purchasing this book!

I hope this book was able to help you to better understand the different benefits that using body butter regularly can provide you with. At the same time, we also hope that you're able to gain the information you need to get started with making some of your own, using all natural ingredients and right in the comfort of your own home.

The next step is to give any of the recipes provided a try. They are easy to follow and the ingredients you'll need are widely available, not to mention safe enough for your kids to use them as well. This way, the whole family can partake in your projects and be able to enjoy the products you're able to make as well. Give them out as gifts or if you have the entrepreneurial spirit, turn it into a small business.

With just a bit of imagination, anything is possible!

In addition, please remember to check out our Facebook page in order to find other resources and upcoming promotions:

https://www.facebook.com/joypublishing

With sincere thanks,

EVA HUNTER

One **Last** *Thing...*

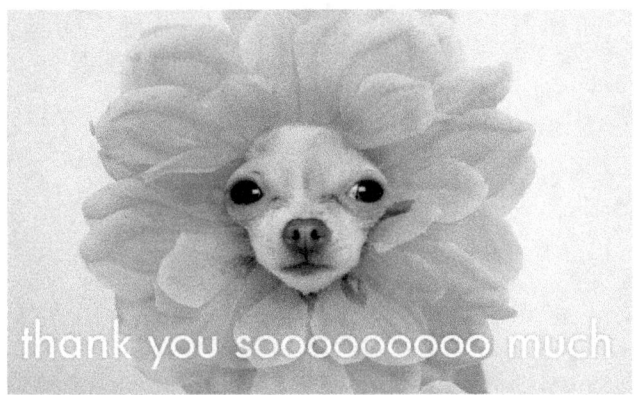

Source: Wikipedia

If you believe that this book is worth sharing, would you please take the time to let others know how it affected your life? If it turns out to make a difference in the lives of others, they will be forever grateful to you, as will I.

www.ingramcontent.com/pod-product-compliance
Lightning Source LLC
Chambersburg PA
CBHW060443290526
45793CB00002B/558